WORTHY BEAUTY

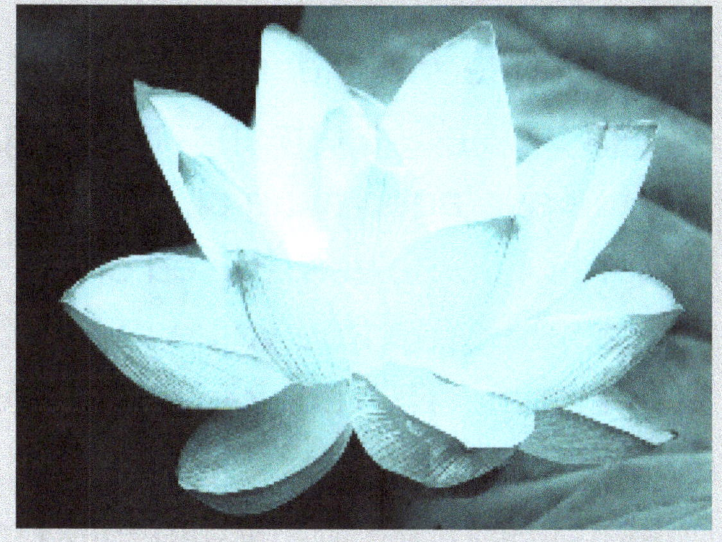

Subtitle: Mother & Daughters of Grace

For Ages 10 and up.

By:Wisdom Palm El Bey

Introduction

This book is for young teens, older adults, and those who just want to accept the knowledge that is being provided. This book gives the average young or older woman the reason to take care of ourselves. Based on true scientific facts, this book captures the true value of an ageless woman and their stories. This book is meant to give women like me the idea to respect and protect what is valued as a human being. Also keep in mind that it is a bliss to know this knowledge that is being provided, and is essentially phenomenal without a curse. I would like to thank all those who shared their true stories with me, to all my readers, mentors, editors, and publishers, and all the wonderful people that delivered for me it is truly an honor. Thank you for your patient, for your experience is the true reason why this book will always stay alive because you alone give breath to the knowledge of the known and unknown. Thank you creator of all things I give the honor first to thee.! Peace and love to all!

TABLE OF CONTENTS:

CHAPTER 1

What I didn't know!

The day I turned 13 was the day I decided to wear white to school. One of the most beautiful and important days of my life because it was the day that I would soon be a teenager. I waited so long, it seemed for this day, I called my birthday, was finally here. I was so excited because being a teen means closer to being an adult and even though I liked boys, I was not sure if I wanted or even needed a boyfriend. However, what I was for sure about was looking good while going to school, cause that was when appearance really mattered, hygiene and all. For a teenager, it is hard being somewhere to belong or even being in the right place in life. Out of all those worries, something even bigger than ever came as a surprise on my birthday and that was called the red dot (period) in my beautiful white that represented me as pure light. Not anymore! Because there was a red dot in the back of my pants. Take Laura for instance she started when she was 10 years old on the playground at recess. She had to run in the girl's bathroom in a panic, and she said she used the whole tissue roll. When she got home she ran to the back and her sister told her what to do. However, what her sister didn't tell her was how to put them on. So poor Laura was putting pads on backward. She, 'said' she felt so ashamed that she had isolated herself at school. Back to my story. How embarrassing, frustrated, and painful, and most of all angry I was with my experience! I could only imagine how poor Laura had felt. There were no instructions that told me not to wear my beautiful white at all. My mother told me a little about what to do if it happened. However she didn't mention the cramps it brings, how to remedy the painful situation, stress, warning signs, or the real price that I alone will go through to take care of my body. She probably didn't tell me because she didn't know herself, no blame on her behavior but knowledge is power. The real cost to support a woman's menstruation is priceless yet expensive in today's world. This book is for people like me or people who just may not have the type of guardian in their life. Living in today's world of 2020 this could be troubling times, for most people. For those of you who just need to get your mind at ease or wish to learn more remedies then this book is for you as well. So here are a few pointers on how to remedy the red dot. If you are suffering from the red dot, also known as...our period, then you're not alone. More likely your body is changing, changing into beautiful lovely energy. So that means your body is experiencing an imbalance of nature, some call it 'The earthquake'. Your body hormones start to rise even more and you may have thought you didn't care for boys, but you find yourself hanging out with a crew of girls crushing on a crew of boys. What a coincidence. Here it is you got the red dot going on, hormones racing, and you're bleeding on yourself for five to seven days out of the month, every month of 365 days of the year! There just got to be some kind of remedy for the stress, depression and the pain just got to be! Well, in my day the knowledge I'm about to tell you was not provided to me in the way that I am about to prescribe

to you. So all this great kool-aid I'm about to spill, get ready for this A and B conversation so C
your way in! (Ok that was horrid)

CHAPTER 2

Remedies for the red dot

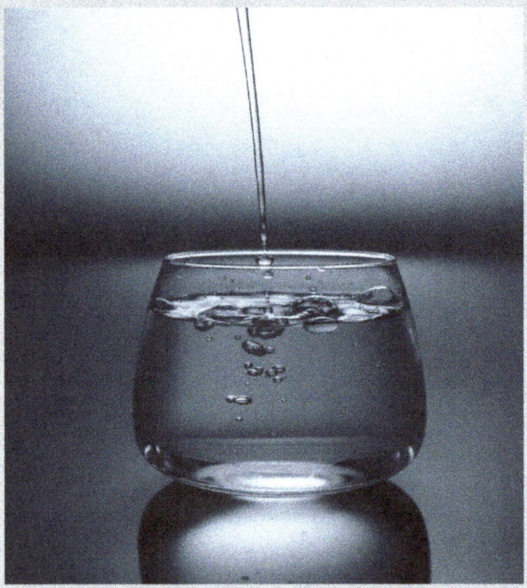

(1.) Water, drink plenty of clean purified 8oz of water to reduce pain, and to balance out your body, a study has shown that water alone creates memory as well 90% of our body is made of water. Water can help with back pain and other illnesses that may occur.

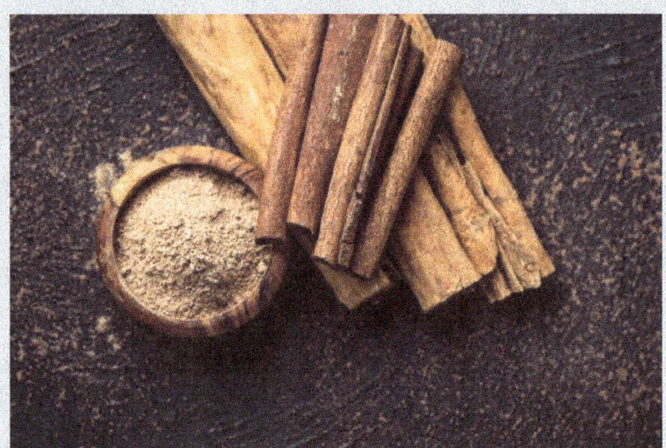

(2.) Cinnamon 1 teaspoon and 1 teaspoon cayenne pepper with a touch of peppermint and some honey, taste very good and good for the soul.

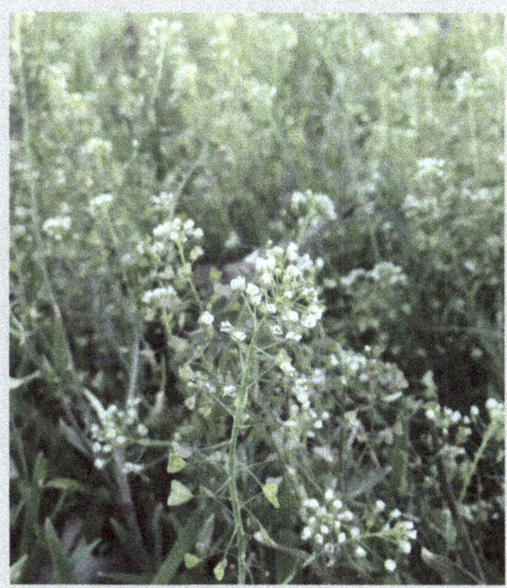

(3.) Shepherd purse also is known as Capsella bursa - pastries is a plant base flower that is good for headache, vomiting, blood in your urine, diarrhea, and bladder infection women use shepherd's purse for the menstrual cramp to reduce the amount of time you're on your red dot. Superficial burns and skin injuries are the side effects you may ask the answer is yes and no. Too much of anything can kill you however a shepherd purse is safe as long as you don't overdose that is a fact. Make it as a tea with 1 teaspoon of honey.

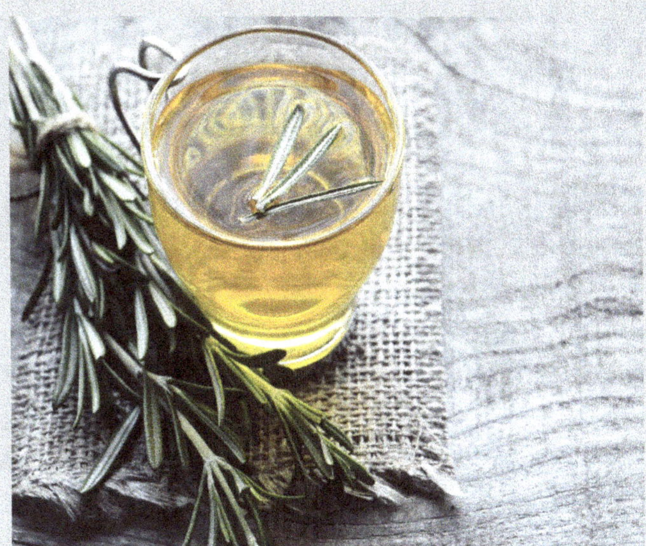

(4.) Rosemary is a bitter herb. Rosemary was traditionally used to help muscle spazz, memory loss, and traditionally boost the immune system, circulatory system and promote hair growth as a stimulant plant.

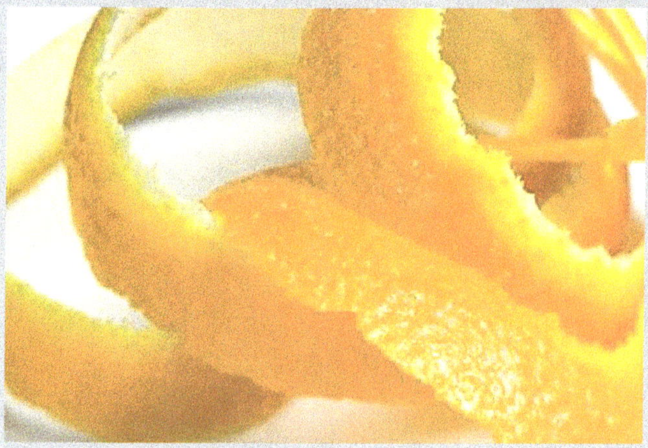

(5.) Orange peeling: Orange peels have vitamin C and contain 136 mg of vitamin C. It is also replete with copper calcium magnesium folate vitamin A and vitamin B and dietary fibers. Best nutrition contributes to the human body.

  Orange peelings can be used for your menstrual, to lower your blood pressure, for eczema and depression, and improve heart health by lowering bad cholesterol. Orange peelings aid in weight loss and respiratory issues. Using orange peelings can help protect you from cancer while preventing digestive issues and heartburn. Other properties that orange peelings can help prevent is improving oral health and freshens up your breath. It helps to aid hangovers. Orange peeling is a great product to use to nurture yourself. With a touch of honey or some sweet milk. You're all good to go. Another thing that was not thought of and I had to find out on my own. There are so many different ways to go about the red dot (period) that you can use and so many pads and tampons that are available for women to use to help with the pain, heavy flowing and to keep your body balanced while you're on your menstrual period. To be honest, to feel good or even normal while on your red dot. The average cost for your personal hygiene, you would need to spend between 100 to 200 dollars on your personal lady product easily. The reason why is because women are very sensitive. Our pearl is priceless yet worth every diamond, ruby, penny, dime, Quarter, and nickel, etc. You could elevate half of that by DIY and making your own products for your simple needs. Really it all depends on how you would like to go about it. First and most it is very important to eat right. Nowadays food is not as real as it used to be, It is all fake so it is very important to research your food. Not just for your health but for you to keep your menstrual red dot under control and balance.

CHAPTER 3

Different tampons and pads.

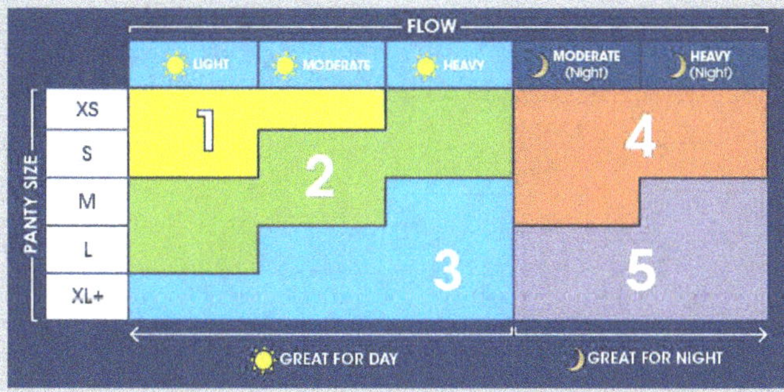

There are a variety of different pads and tampons you can use. There are chlorine-based tampons and pads cotton base tampons and pads made out of the fiber, tampons, and pads made out of cotton cloth. Really it all depends on how you want to go about the fit and the comfort. When choosing a pad you want to look for pads that do not cause irritation and long-lasting pads that absorb for a number of hours. Also, it is important that you know what is going in and out of your VJ (vagina). This chapter describes and tells you the best and not so best pads to use for your essentials and also the danger that causes issues with your VJ (vagina).

Tips to know!: Ladies, there's multiple bacterias and BV alone that can cause your vajayjay to go raw, and to go out of balance. So it is very important to take care of your vajayjay. Here are a few tips that you can do.

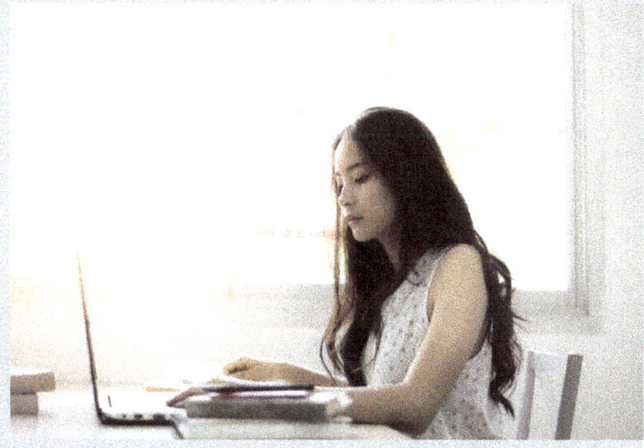

(1.) Research all of the products that you want to use for your menstruation. Because it is very important to know what your body needs and what it can handle.

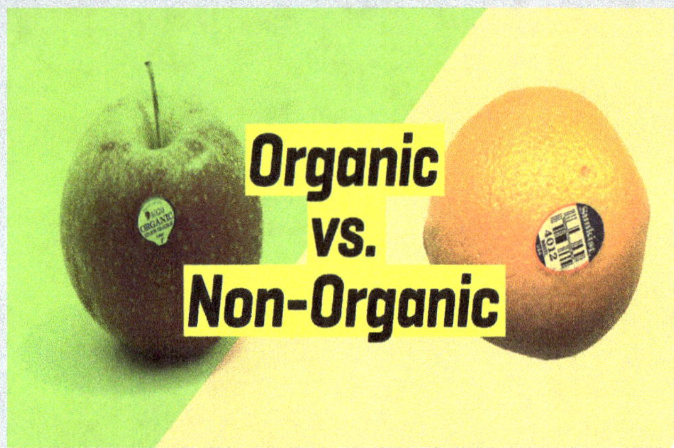

(2.) Decide if you're going organic or non-organic

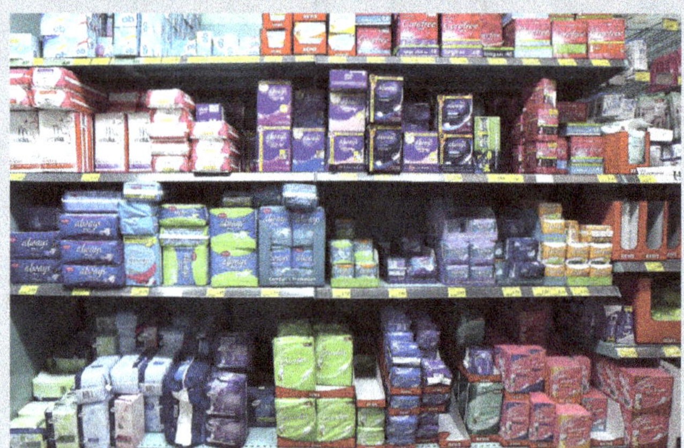

(3.) Try out different products and brands so you have a backup plan in case the brand you're using goes out of business.

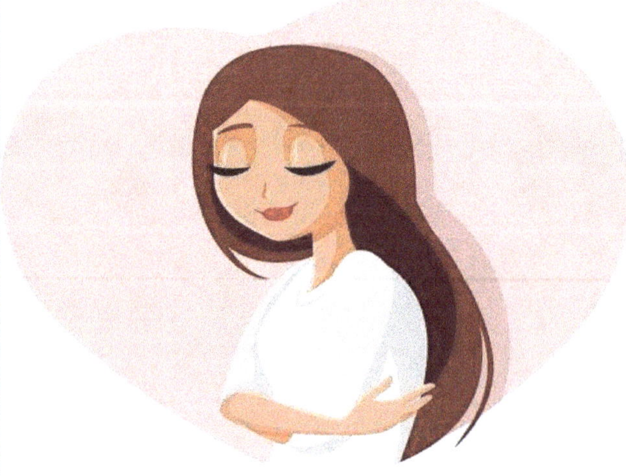

(4.) Don't be afraid of your body.

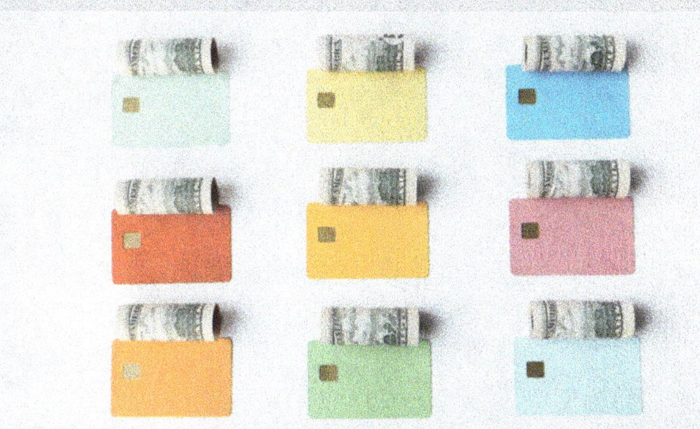

(5.) Plan your budget even though it is expensive to take care of your vjj. You can learn to budget while having the best quality ever.

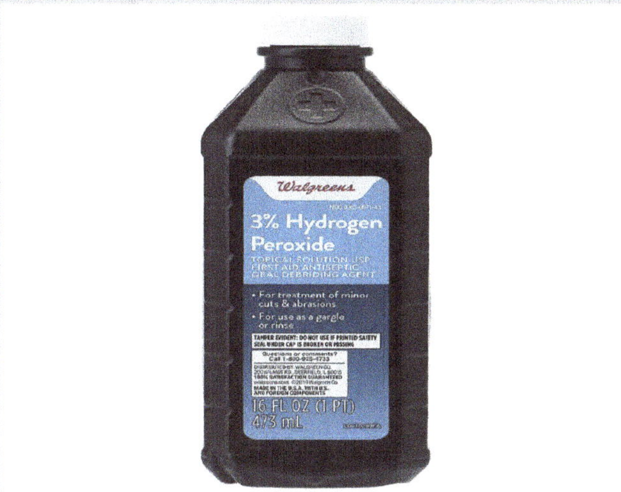

(6.) You may use hydrogen peroxide 3%. Use as a douche to treat bv and yeast infection, however, always ask your doctor for recommendations. To start to dilute half peroxide and half water normal like a douche.

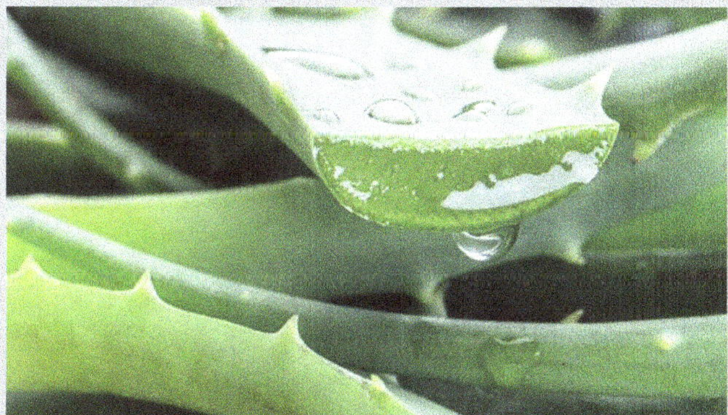

(7.) Aloe vera is good to get rid of B.V (Bacterial Vagal Infection) applied on the skin as a lotion or cream.

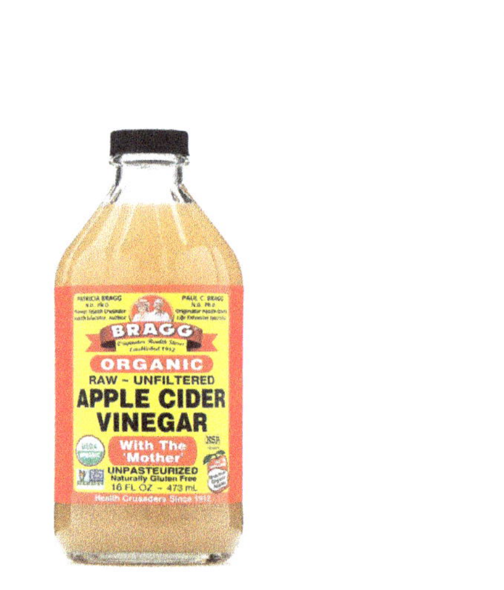

(8.) Apple cider vinegar gets rid of bv or yeast infection There are three ways to use this recipe. First, you could use as a douche by felling a douche bottle half with water and half with apple cider vinegar or you could dip a tampon by soaking for 2 to 3 mins in apple cider vinegar and inserting the tampon leave in your vajayjay for 2 to 4 hours. repeat for 2 days straight. Or you could soak your body in a bathtub.

9.) Borax soap can be used for B.V or yeast infection. There Is a soap already made to use or you can dilute a pinch or teaspoon of borax soap and put in bath water every 5-gallon tub of water. You don't need a lot of borax soap. Soak your body in water. Do this for three days and you are good to go. **Make sure it says** 'Borax Bath Soap'.

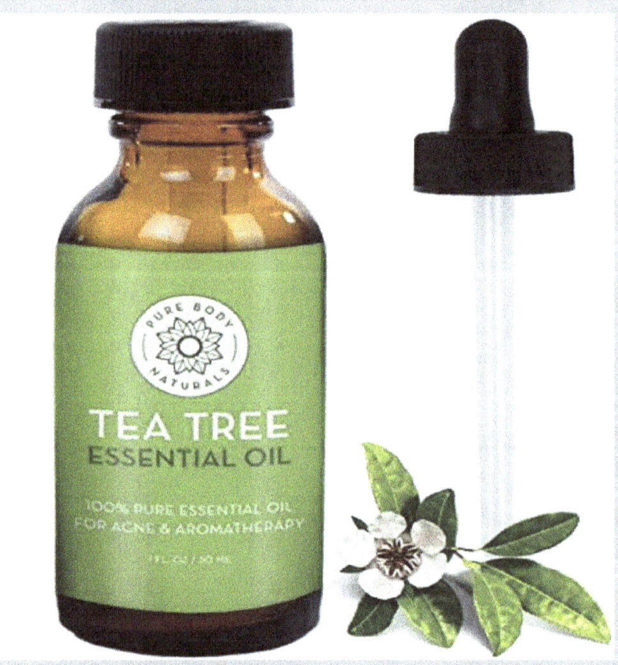

(10.) Tea tree oil is one of the most all-purpose oils ever used. All essential oils should be diluted with water or carrier oil for bv. Make it into a spray soak on a tampon used as a cream.

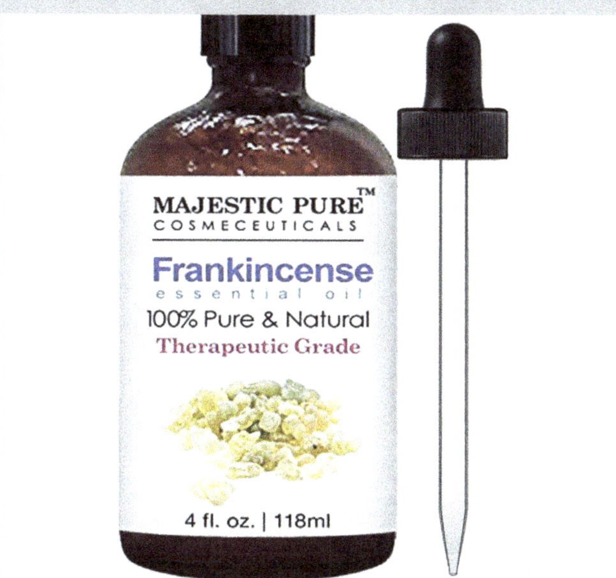

(11.) Frankincense is very good for bv yeast infection.

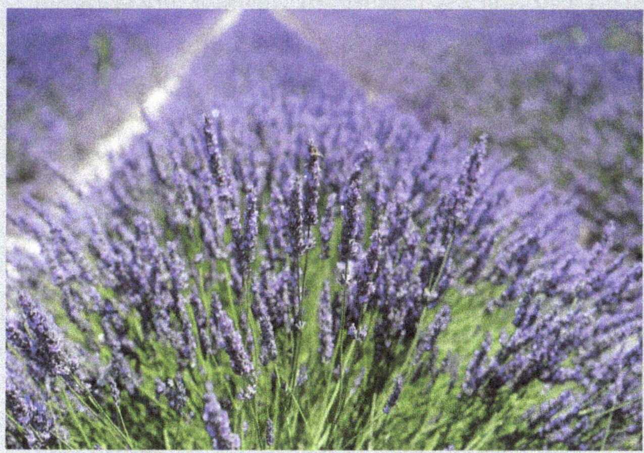

(12.) lavender could be used for yeast and B.V.

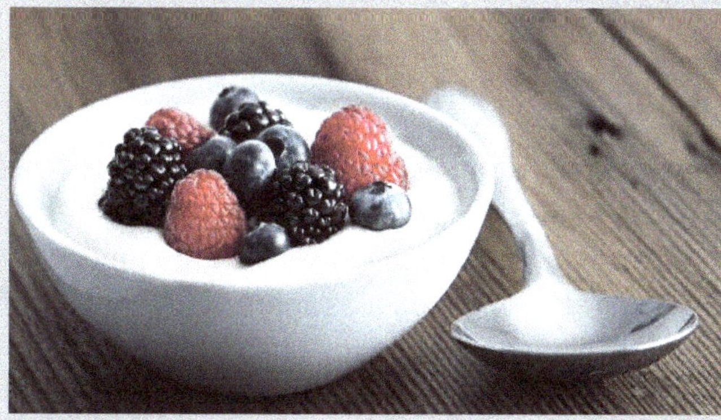

(13.) Eat yogurt that can help you get rid of bv or yeast infections.

The study has shown that eating more green food and less meat can help your body during the menstrual process to flow lighter and easy flow. (Harvard University.)

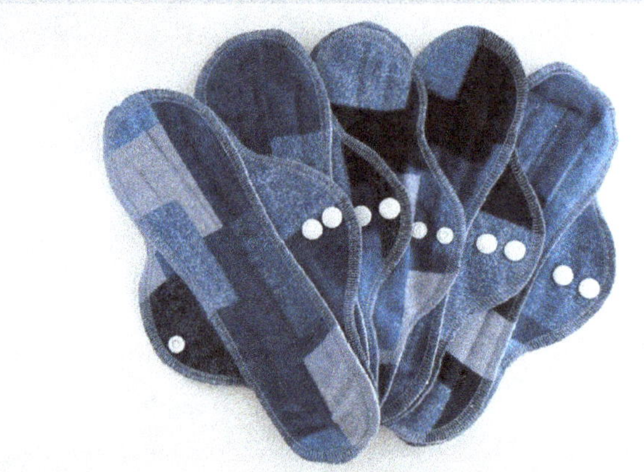

   The two types of pads that are made are called external and internal: one goes inside of your vagina and one goes on the outside of your vagina. Only you know your body and know what is comfortable. Ladies, I can't stress the fact that you have to get to know your cookie and love yourself. Loving yourself is loving your cookie. The key point is trusting in yourself while loving yourself, is loving the god in you. Everything after that will become valued as follows. Back to the subject. There's only two that you can pick internally that are not for sensitive people or should I say sensitive skin. However, when choosing, you should choose something that's organic or non-organic. If you choose to go on long trips you can use cloth pads that are washable. That would be the best choice even though it sounds gross for the moment; however, it is your blood, your body, you have nothing to be ashamed about. It is perfectly natural. Cloth pads are the best and the safest. There are sponge pads as well that are made from sea material however some say it is safe, some say it is not! If I was you I wouldn't take the chance. However, a lot of doctors don't know about this kind of pads being used so do your research. There are a lot of chlorine base pads and other chemicals in pads that you should be aware of. According to the National Center for research study showed that there is some discomforting news about the chemical being exposed to women's bodies. So products **ALWAYS** have chemicals in their pads, Kotex they as well. DON'T PANIC! There are others that you can use such as Kotex ultra-thin pads, Laloa pads, and tampons. Maxi pads, diva cups, jade sea sponges, the carefree anti-free seventh-generation. There are even organic tampons that put your body back on balance. So if you bleed real heavy or very long like seven days long some of the organic pads and tampons can change the directions of things. Let's talk a little about panty liners. Pantyliners are a lady's friend. It is a little pad-like but is much thinner and lighter for women when they're just getting off their red dot (period) or discharging. There are four different brands to consider like Poise, Un Kotex, carefree thongs, panties liners, and more. Use panties liners for light flow, never heavier flow. Panties liners are not pads but a great helper for pads and a way to keep your underclothes cleaner. The best advice I can tell you is to research your product because it is well worth the knowledge.

CHAPTER 4

Can you use soap on your vajayjay?

  I guess the question that is asked by young ladies and women is can you use soap or body wash on your vagina and if so, is it safe. The answer to that particular question is very complicated yet can be answered with a satisfaction guarantee. You can use soap on the vajayjay. However, it does not mean that it is not a risky business. Not to mention that soap that is used on your vajayjay can cause yeast infections and B.V. However, it all depends on who made the soap and if the soap is generally made to help ph balance in your vajayjay.
Soap clogs up the pores in our body and in that particular sensitive area in our vagina. Also, some soap can cause burning sensations, itching, and irritation of the skin. So make sure you read the ingredients on the soap. It is very good to learn to make your own soap for your own personal self. That knowledge can go a long way. There is a variety of soap to choose from like Aveeno fragrances free bar soap, Neutrogena, Eucerin, summer eve, Queen V soap, Yoni washes for vegan and yes of course dove unscented soap there is much more while I am only naming a few. Ladies, let's face it, who wants to walk around smelly all day? I sure don't! it is not ladylike.

CHAPTER 5

Washing powder & Detergent

   It is my heart's desire to discuss how important it is to use the right washing powders and detergents when it comes to your red dot (period). You must be very sanitary when messing around with blood, it is an important factor in your health and others. To prevent harm to yourself or someone else, here are a few key tips that can help you stay sanitized while on your red dot. When washing your underclothes you want to make sure that your underclothes are meeting the requirements; and that is fresh scented and most of all a clean feeling. The best washing powder to use for the menstrual period is Clorox color-safe detergent, Baking soda Arm & hammer, Borax laundry detergent, or powder with some peroxide mix with it because you are dealing with blood and odors. You need to wash your underclothes out by hand first then rinse then wash in the washing machine. You may want to wear plastic gloves when touching blood even if it is yours. Squeezing lemon on your area to remove hard spots that may be tough to get out is a good tip you may want to consider. Let your underclothes sit for about 30mins in a container that you use just for your personal needs. Water than hand wash and rinse clean your area with some type of disinfectant and you will be good to go. Disinfectants you may use is Lysol, bleach, fabulous, or you may not want to use chemicals that can harm you so you could use lemons, orange, vinegar, witch hazel rubbing alcohol, sage spray, tea tree oil spray anything that kills germs feel free to use at your own risk. As a younger or older lady, you want to feel clean and fresh while smelling good. Not to mention it is important to keep yourself intact so you don't get sick.

CHAPTER 6

Panties to wear while on your menstrual

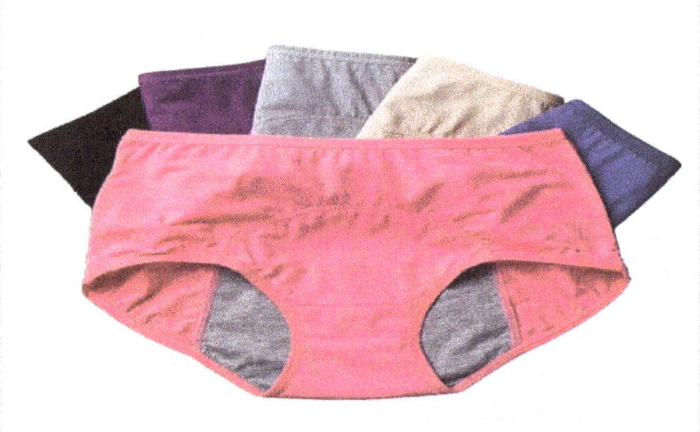

There is a variety of underwear that can support you on your red dot (period). Wearing the right kind of underwear is almost to your essential natural condition. There are companies that make such comfortable underwear that can assist with the comfort and controlling of your day, making it so much easier for you when the time of the month comes. Companies like RUBY LOVE, THINX, MODI BODI, DEAR KATE, YOYI FASHION, and RAEL, just to name a few and there is so much more to choose from. One of my favorite kinds is called CUPID GIRDLE UNDERWEARS, these underwears are good to use and hold pads or tampons in place. There is nothing more convenient than to know that you are in a comfortable state of mind and in doing so you can look and feel good all at the same time. The next chapter is a whole new world of life! We will be talking about our face and what to do to keep it looking younger and healthier. You will learn some of the best beauty secrets that you ever came across. So sit back and enjoy a reader's wealth and remember taking care of you is what matters at the end of the day.

CHAPTER 7

Taking care of your face

Taking care of your face is not just an essential but the fact that you can stop time in its place is really what's important. To do so it is a very important key aspect of how to do just that. Starting from a young lady you have the baby skin and the right glow that is so appealing to others. Getting your skin to stay like a baby is a challenge. Did you know that once you are conceived from your mother's womb you are getting older? Your telomeres, which are your DNA cells from structural molecules, are aging you as soon as you hit the air. The strands of your telomeres are long at birth but when you age they start to get shorter which causes you to look older than you appear. So once you are born you're dying.

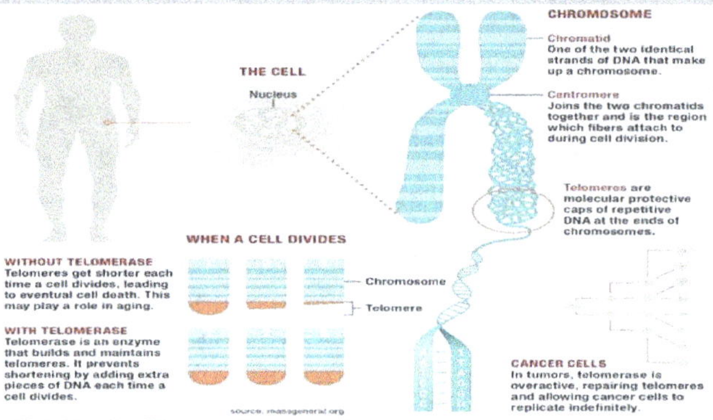

Most people got it all wrong. They say after a certain age your body starts to give out and you start to look older than dust. Maybe that part of that fact is true if you don't take care of your body. Because if you don't take care of your body then there's just a matter of time, your telomerase DNA line will get shorter and you will see results of old age quickly and fast and you will start to deteriorate rapidly. You'd be lucky if your bones won't start to decay. Most older women begin to get in panicky attacks around their thirties or so maybe even the forties. They try to find what works because it is a process in the making. So with that said," in general, it does take time and patience to accumulate a positive health effect, younger-looking skin tone, skin complexion or beauty you're looking for as you age slowly. I am here to give you the facts ladies and gentlemen, no discrimination going on in my book, so let's get started.

CHAPTER 8

Washing your face

  Washing your face with just some cold water can be a huge step to a very beautiful skin complexion. However, because the water has fluoride it could be damaging to your skin and body. So if you want clean unpolluted skin tone it is best to clean your face with the most purity. So with all respect that is why facial cleaning soaps and sprays are made. You can make your own if you are crafty or, you can buy from professionals that are on the market. In the meantime get yourself a really good cleanser that could help you on your goals to healthier-looking skin. There are a lot of different brands such as Cetaphil, LaRoche Hydrating, Ceveve, B3, Clinique cleansing balm, Pacifica Sea Foam, and plenty more just to name a few. When washing your face with cleansers be sure to leave on for 10 to 15 minutes then wash off the face. Never leave overnight unless directed. Then you can apply your cream or moisturizer, serum, or cream for a toner. All the brands that are described are great face washes to use for your skin, some for poor skin, acne pro, blackheads, whiteheads, wrinkles, etc. You name it, that is the true fact that a dermatologist would recommend that it is FDA APPROVED. However, there are other essentials that can be used like honey and lemon in which case can be used to remove unwanted freckles and sunburn.

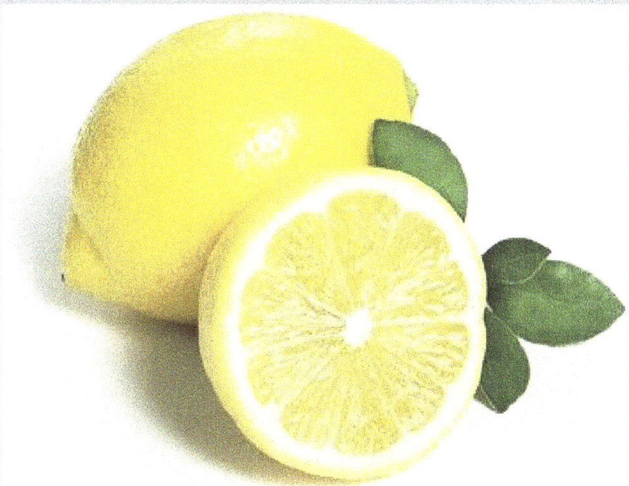

(1.) Lemons as you may or may not know is a acid citric antioxidant, antifungal natural vitamin C it can help aid in acne, blackheads, pimples, you name it, it will be done it can even aid in lighting up your skin or lighting up dark spots like freckles. Lemon can be drunk as water and can also be used as an essential oil. Lemon is a good one to use for your face as well. Use a touch of olive oil to give a good tone and rosy cheeks.

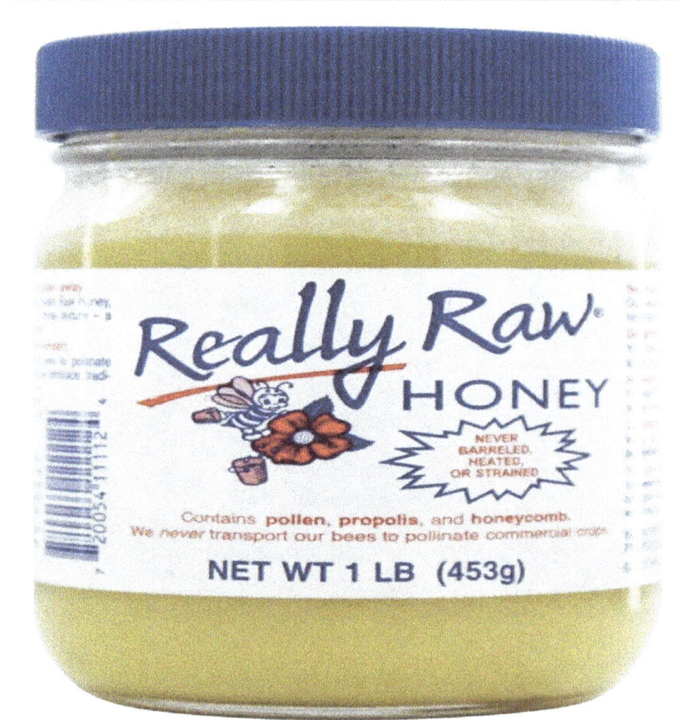

(2.) Honey can be used to remove scars, burn marks or any first or second third-degree burns just be sure to apply every night until you are satisfied with your results. Honey benefits and properties are rich in antioxidants it can increase your blood flow, fight off unwanted infection. The best type of honey to use is raw honey because the impurities have better healing effects.

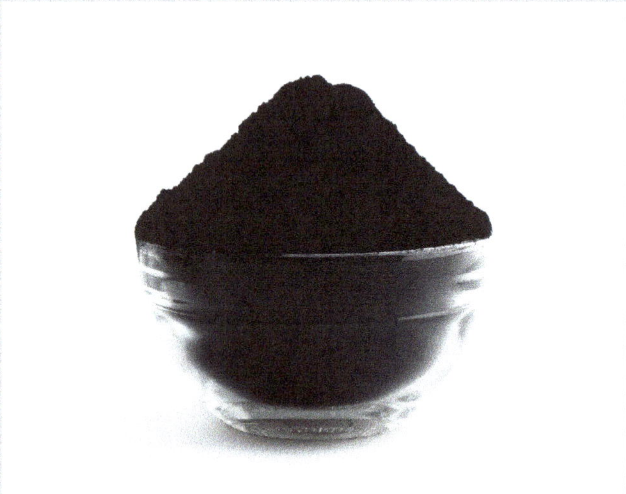

(3.) Activated charcoal is great as it is a detoxification and digestion healer that kills any bacteria that you may come across in your life. You can use activated charcoal as a face mask to help with blackheads.

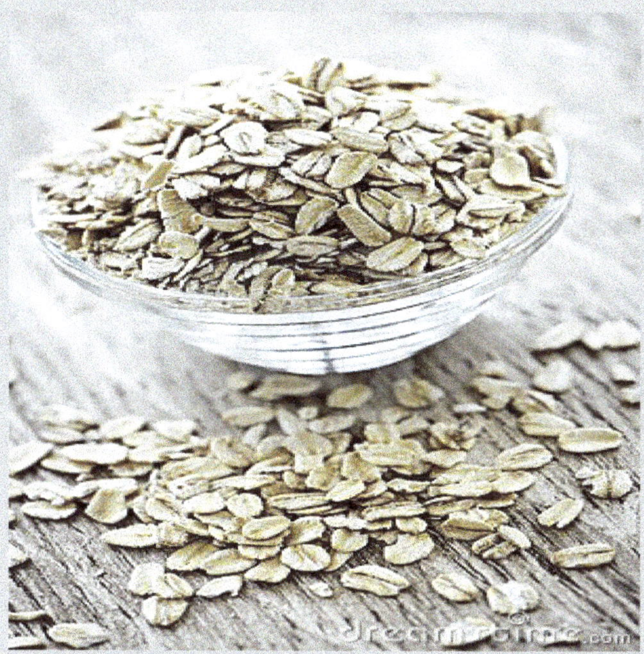

(4.) Oatmeal face wash treatment can treat it has antioxidants and anti-inflammatory properties it also helps with dry skin. Oatmeal oat as saponin compounds that are natural cleansers. Clogs dirt oils even any irritation on your skin can be solved with the use of oatmeal face wash.

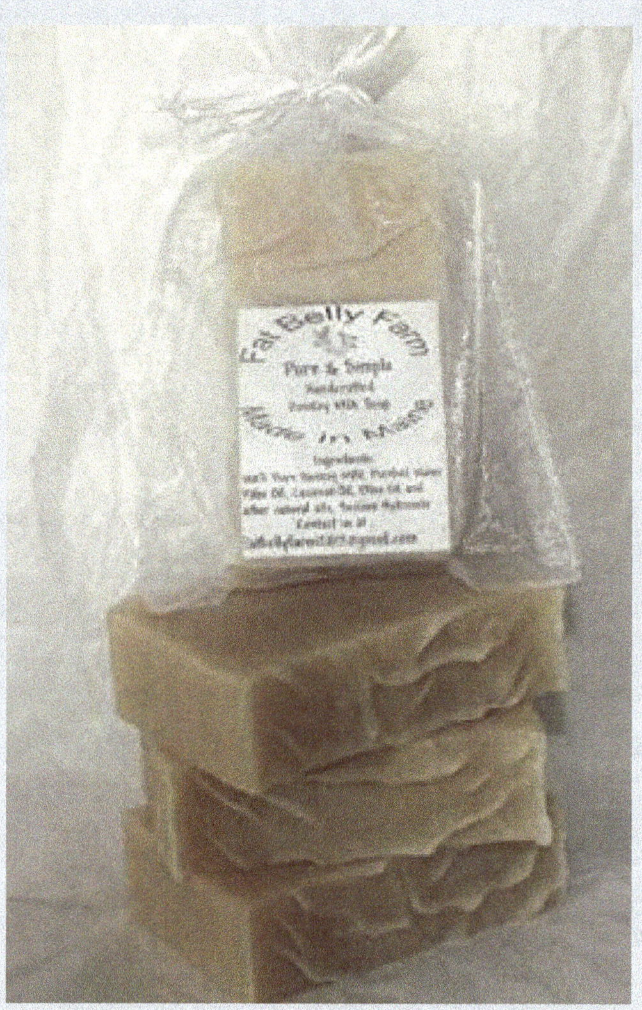

(5.) My favorite one of a kind that Cleopatra used was donkey milk soap. Her beauty secret was and still is a hit and a dashing phenomenal! She used real donkey milk on her face and even bathed in the milk from time to time. Leaving her skin young and radiant. Donkey milk is a fatty acid with Omega-3, its minerals, and vitamins of A, B1, B2, B6, D, AND, E according to donkeymilkbeauty.com. Donkey milk also contains vitamin c and is lactose with a touch of casein with this, said using donkey's milk as a face soap not only can leave your skin healthy and looking beautiful but can regenerate the skin cells. No wonder why Cleopatra was so beautiful.!

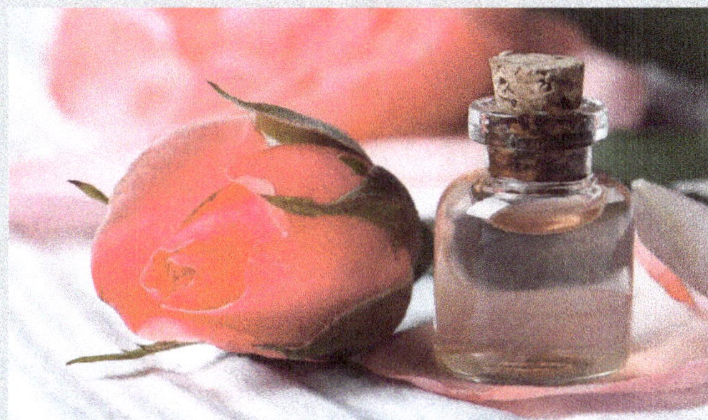

(6.) Another facewash secret is rosewater. Rosewater is great for your skin and is a natural toner for your face it can and well help you stay in a ph balance, keep control of irritation, and is an anti-inflammatory product with vitamins of A, B3, C, D and, E supporting its values. You can't go wrong with rosewater.

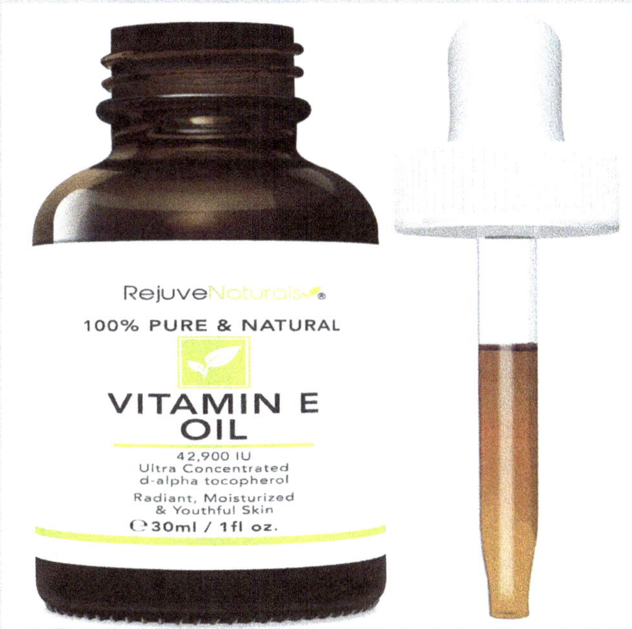

(7.) vitamin E as we all know that applying vitamin E to your skin can leave your skin looking healthy and full along with you getting good looking skin.

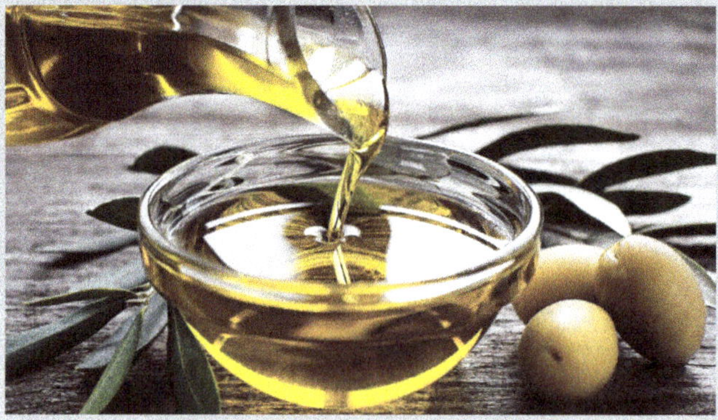

(8.) Almond oil. Now I love almond oil. It is one of the best antioxidants inflammatory oils that I ever came across for your skin. It has Vitamin E inside oil along with vitamins A and d and B that supports the skin In a major way leaving your skin looking and feeling immaculate and straight beautiful.

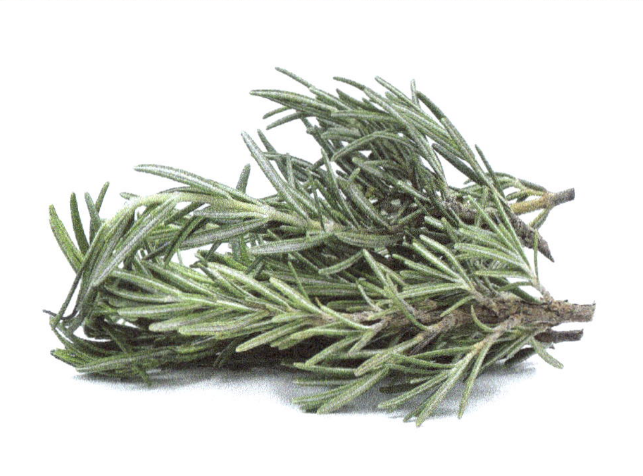

(9.) Rosemary: Rosemary is not only a stimulant for your nerves in your face but is a great toner leaving your skin looking flawless!

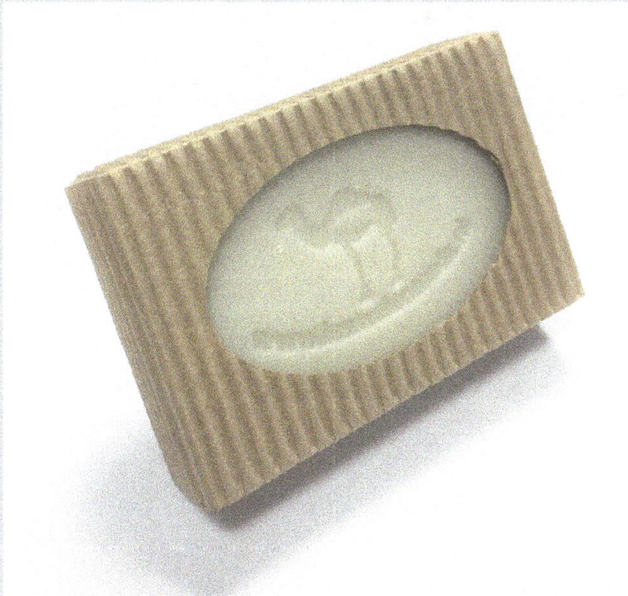

(10.)My number one best secret ever is camel milk soap. Yes, camel milk! Camel milk is one of the best milk ever known and the closest to human breast milk you could never go wrong it is an antioxidant compound that regenerates dead cells and renews as well you will look younger for sure with this milk. Camel milk can remove dark marks, blemishes, pigmentation issues, acne, and more. Not too many people know about this secret!. If you can get your hands on these milk ladies, you're in the game.!

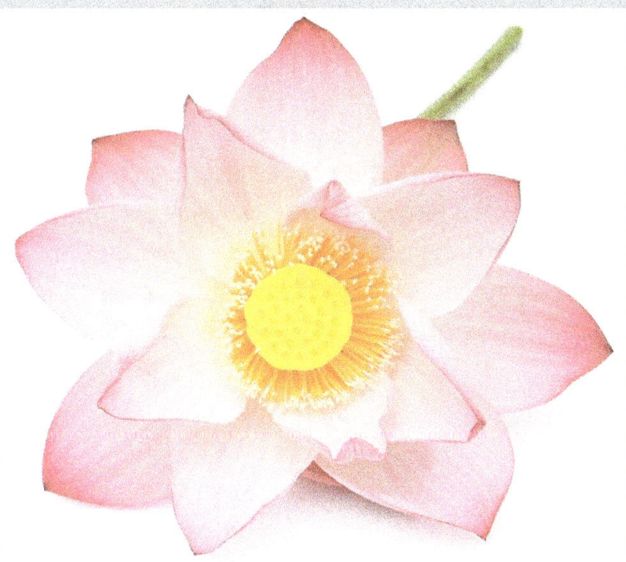

(11.) I guess I will give you one more of my secrets: one of the best,.That is the Lotus flower oil get your hand on some of this and you are the peaches and the cream. The lotus flower is a flower that comes in different colors and each color has different properties that can be used for your skin, your hair, even your health. The Lotus flower can regenerate and rebuild your immune system. That means not a cure but by remedy cancer killer effect. Take caution not to use lotus flowers while pregnant because there is not enough evidence to show that the lotus flower can cause irritation to your baby. I could go on, but I will not! That will be the end of this CHAPTER let's save some secrets for my next book cause we just getting warmed up on the juice I got to give.

CHAPTER 9

Exercising facial muscles

From the time you enter this world as a baby to a child, teen, young adult, to middle age to old age all that time is the first time your body starts to age as quickly as you were born. It is important to learn to slow the process down. It really doesn't matter how young or old you are either way it goes. You're going to age but it is up to you to control the way you look, feel, and process. One way by doing that without any soap, lotion, creams, the serum is by exercising your face. So you can exercise a certain part of your face like your chin and control an overlap of a double chin you may have developed over the years as you age. You can exercise your jaw and cheekbones to get a natural facelift. You can help to stop aging by developing muscle in your face. You can defeat crow feet and early rankles by building your cells and rejuvenate the process of aging skin by face exercising. The method is an easy yoga, Ayurveda approach, or simply an ancient Chinese method that you could use. This method is science beyond your years that our ancestors carried out for the generations. It is important to remember where you come from. So you can know where you are going in life. To slow your age down is an important factor that is well appreciated. I am glad to share this information with you and I hope that now that I have mentioned a few good pointers to you now you can manage the rest by researching the facts on your own. Read books and look up on youtube on ways to exercise your face for a healthier-looking ageless younger skin.

Why face exercises?:
Face yoga is one of the ancient methods that our ancestors used to keep a healthy-looking skin. By exercising the muscles in your face you can slow or even stop the aging process in your face and look 10 times younger. Because there are so many facial poses that you could consider from different backgrounds of religion my niece will demonstrate some of these exercises so you will know what to do.

Pose 1

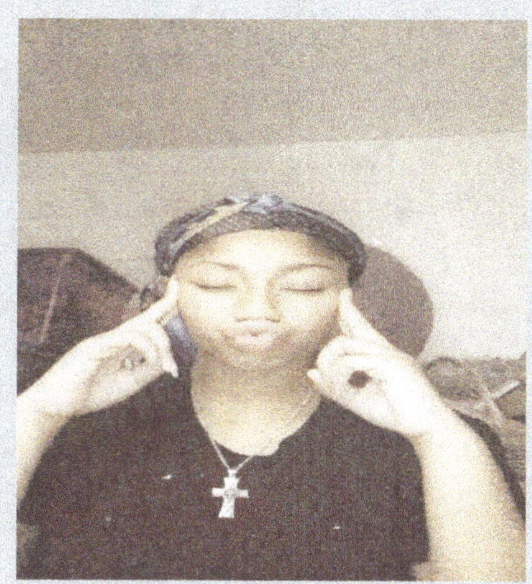

Pose 2

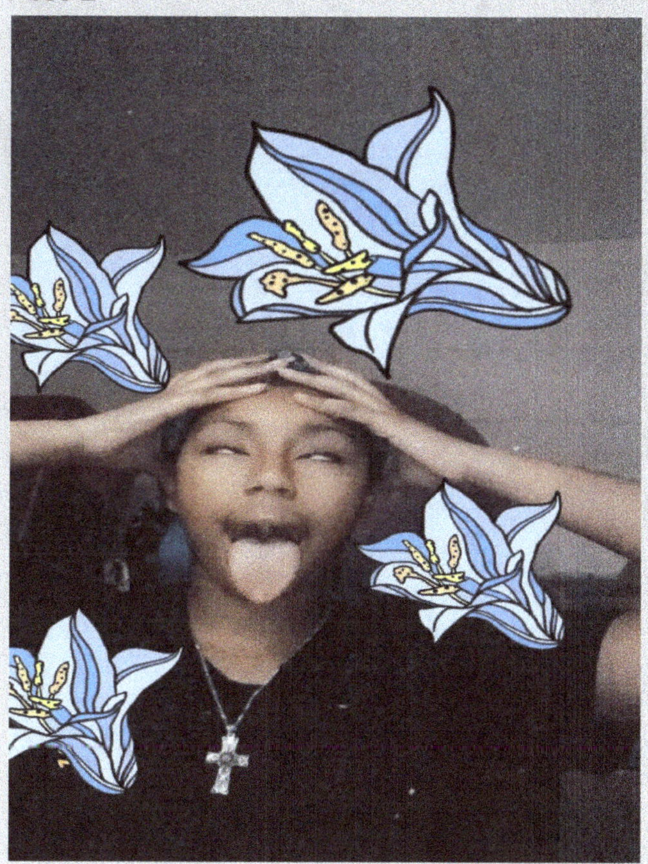

Pose 3

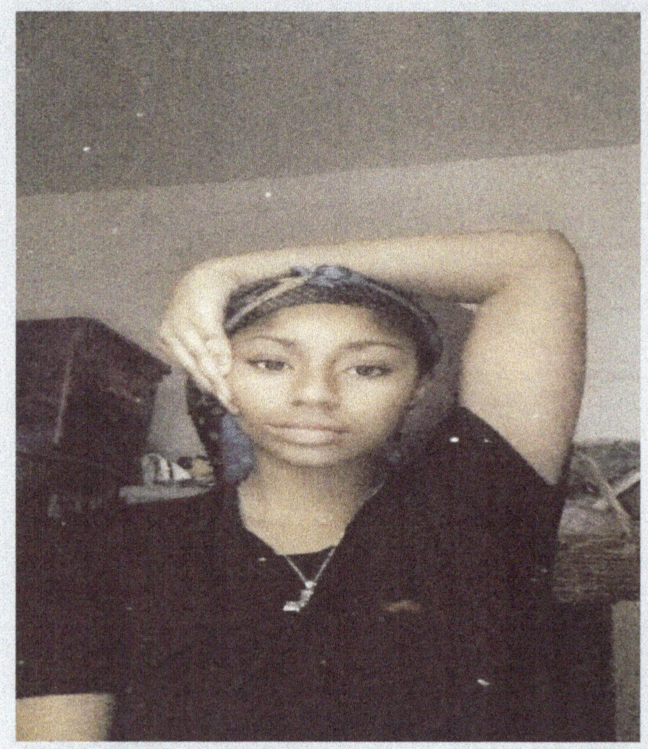

Pose 4

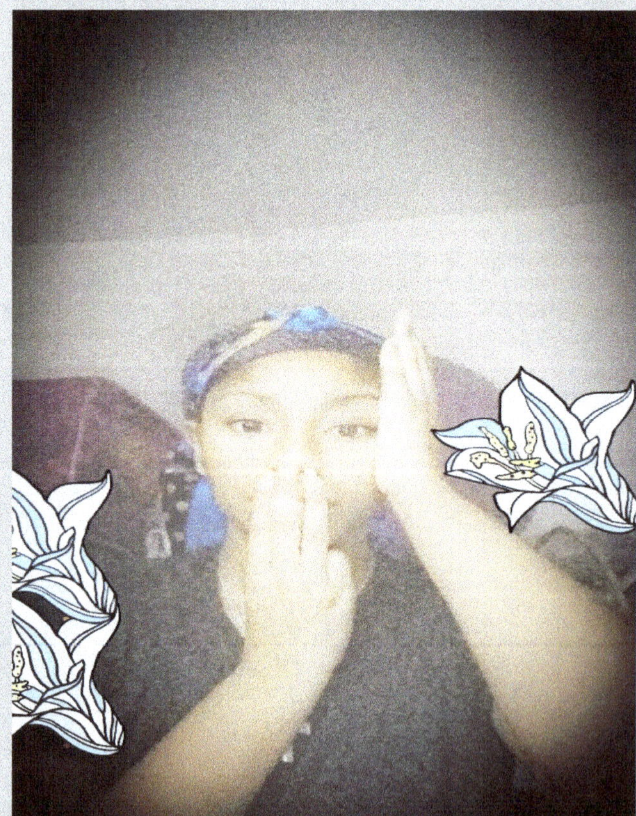

Pose 5

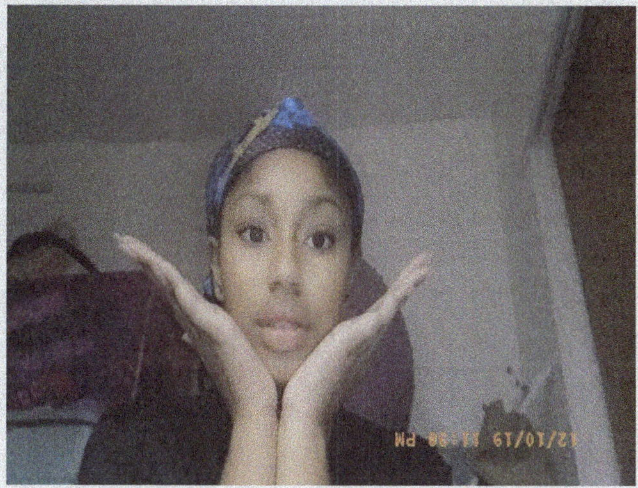

However, my job in this book is to give you the great news that you can discover when doing your own research. Next in chapter 10, we will discuss The value and the process of growing your hair. So have fun reading this chapter.

CHAPTER 10

The summary of hair

   The hair on the head and on the body has always had history and value to its story. Some ancient people in some religions believed that hair is considered one of the most valuable and important assets of all time. The history behind hair has so many unexplainable capabilities that no scientist still can not explain the power behind its origin. Some ancient cultures believed that hair was considered the alien antenna of the human body and mind. In the King James 611 virgin bible and a matter of fact, all after made bibles Samson was all man with hair that represented his brute strength. In Egypt hair for women was represented in all ways and headcovers like wings and braids. For men in Egypt boldness was a reputation for cleanings and sanitation factors. Knowing your hair texture is very important. The reason is so you can assist your hair with full protection, potential, and greater ability. There are different hair types such as straight hair known as A, wavy hair known by A, B, C, hair type, and curly hair A, B, C type of hair. Research your type of hair so you can manage your hair in a better structure. In the next few chapters, I will be demonstrating exactly just that.

CHAPTER 11

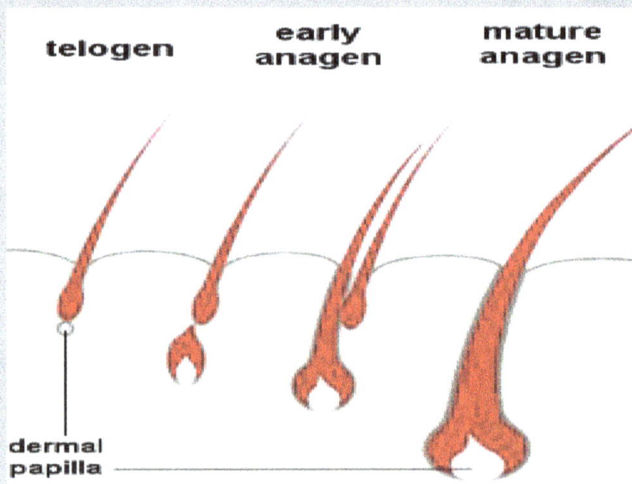

  As you know hair is one of the main essentials of your life. It grows by the root of a bottom follicle. Cells from that follicle are provided by the blood. Your hair has its own protein that it produces naturally and so there it is where your hair begins to grow. However, there are three main stages your hair goes through during its process of growing. These are phrases that contribute to longer hair. The phases are called Anagen, Cartagena, and Telogen. These three phases are cycles, when the cycles are finished it rejuvenates, starting all over again. Look at these pictures for the demonstration.

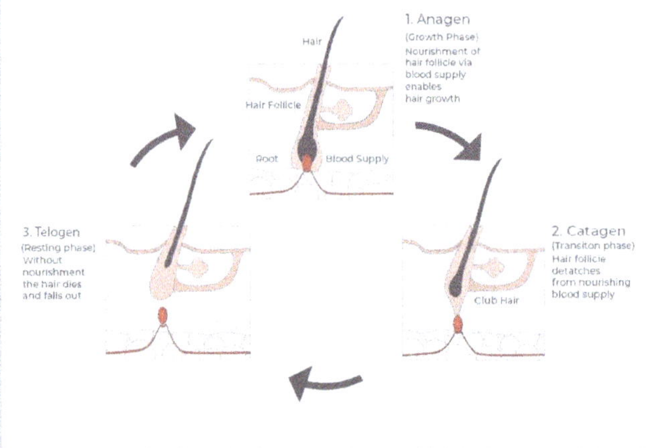

CHAPTER 12

Shampooing the hair

   Shampooing the hair does not only help your hair to grow but it helps you to get rid of unwanted dirt that builds up in your hair follicles. While doing this the process of leaving, your hair feeling good and clean is your result. There are a number of different qualities of shampoo you can use to give your hair a shiny, thick, bounce, there are even powder shampoos. You can make your own shampoo if you know what you are doing. Here is a list of shampoo treatments you can use for your hair. Pantene, Suave, coconut oil shampoo, Jamaican castor oil shampoo, Morocco Macadamia shampoo, Dove shampoo, Pureology shampoo, Garnier Fructis, Tresemme moisturizing shampoo and last but not least, Mane n tail olive shampoo, still one of the best ones that I use. You can even make your own shampoo with the right ingredients that you may like to use. Here is a good recipe you may use for shampoo.

(1.) Start with some donkey milk. This will be one of the most expensive things you make but well worth about 1/4 of a cup. Donkey milk has a rich feature of Omega3 fatty acids and has minerals and nutrients, it is close to DNA milk and one of the best milk ever.

(2.) 1/4 liquid Castile soap, Castile soap good for sensitivity and very safe.

(3.) 20 drops of Rosemary, Rosemary stimulates the hair follicles

(4.) 20 drops of rose oil will give the shine and high-value quality with healing sent.

(5.) 20 drops of carrot oil. Carrot oil has Vitamins such as A to prevent hair loss, strengthens the hair, and also brings blood circulation to your scalp while protecting the root of your hair from pollution.

(6.) One-fourth of a cup of almond oil. Almond oil has Vitamin A, B, D, AND E magnesium, zinc, and potassium, a great benefit of the source to use.

(7.) 40 drops of witch-hazel. Why do witch hazels well? That is to dry the extra unneeded oils that are not needed and to give great circulation as well as scalp treatments.

   Shake well, leave sitting in a dark spot for two days, and continue shaking for the two days, then use, and I bet you got some good shampoo that will last you. If you make a big bottle full it will last for two months, just double the ingredients and you are good to go. Well on the shampoo that is all I will like to give at this time. Let's talk about conditioner masks and hot oil treatments you can use to help your hair to grow or to just simply take care of your hair. As already mentioned, hair is important and it is essential to the human body. Keeping your hair clean by using shampoo can make a big difference. To go the extra mile and give treatment to your hair, you may want to advance by conditioning while putting the mask or hot oil treatments in your hair, this is okay but doing it right is what matters and being safe at all times. You do not want to put too many chemicals in your hair so it's very important that you learn to be more natural because your hair can only take so much however there are people who do perms in their hair, this is by relaxing the hair with a chemical base substance. To be honest there is nothing wrong with doing this. However, if you do it too much you can damage the follicle at the ends and the root of your hair will grow. As a result, heavy damage to your hair and loss can happen. There are some good remedies to do all-natural relaxed hair. I will give you one recipe a little later. Because I want to talk about detanglers. Detanglers are a substance that relaxes the hair which is a leave-in Conditioner. My favorite recipes are 2 tablespoons of apple cider vinegar, 1/4 cup of witch hazel, add some fresh rosemary and some rosemary oil, and some rose oil for scent leave for an hour after you shake. I guarantee you are going to be able to get those hard knots out of your head no matter what. That is the power of detanglers to leave in. There are other good detanglers for your hair especially for type 4 4. Like Aunt Jackie's curls, Kinky-Curly knots and Raw shea butter detangler. There is more than you could imagine. You just have to figure out what is best for your hair type and I can not stress the fact that taking the time to find out will lead to healthier hair.

CHAPTER 13

Treatments for the hair

  Next, let's talk about conditioner and hot oil treatments. Conditioner is a cream that relaxes your hair and moisturizes. It helps keep nutrition in your hair kinda like food for the soul but instead for the hair. There are a lot of different varieties of conditioners out there and so much to pick from it would be impossible to tell you which one works because they all work for different reasons. However, it is always better to pick the one you feel works for you. One of the ones I would recommend to you that I absolutely love is Pantene. I love the shampoo and the conditioner it works well on my type of hair. Now we have talked a little about conditioner, shampoos, and detanglers. Now I want to talk about hot oil treatments. Let's start by talking about what a hot oil treatment is. Hot oil treatment is warmed up oil like almond oil, jojoba oil tea tree oil, or one of my personal favorites that I use every time I make it. Carrot oil is warmed up and placed on the scalp of the head. Why on the scalp, it prevents damage or already damaged hair. It stops the breakage and repair roots of your hair so you will be looking fabulous. To apply hot oil treatment to your scalp simply warm your oil to a decent amount of heat that won't burn you but make you feel warm and tender. Leave in hair for an hour, make sure you wear a hair cap so you don't get oil everywhere. Then wash your hair and condition dry and you are good to go. It is that simple Ladies. Keep in mind that hot oil treatments give your hair, body, and soul back, it has nutrition that is unlocked when heated it also helps your hair to breathe, your hair is going to feel so good ladies, it will be a shame not to do it. Do you want to feel good? Because if you don't you have what they call "issues", and I mean big ones.

CHAPTER 14

Dyeing your hair

  Hair color dyeing goes way back from the Egyptian, Greek, and Roman Times. Hair color is the art of beauty. There are many colors to go from and some of the dyes are plant base. There are Semitic Dyes as well and a mixture of both. Some dyes were made from leeches and walnuts. The reason for hair dyeing is for beauty. HANNA is one of the best natural dyes that is a plant base. It has nutrition and vitamins that are preserved in the plant that helps your hair to grow while providing beautiful color hair. L'oreal is one of the best and still standing in the market. Alma is an Indian herb from India that works great.

CHAPTER 15

Yoga for the hair

 Did you know that you can make your hair grow by doing some hair yoga exercises? Yes! This is a secret that I can not hold back. Here are some demonstrations of a few good poses that you may use to grow your hair long and beautiful.

Pose 1, called downward facing dog.

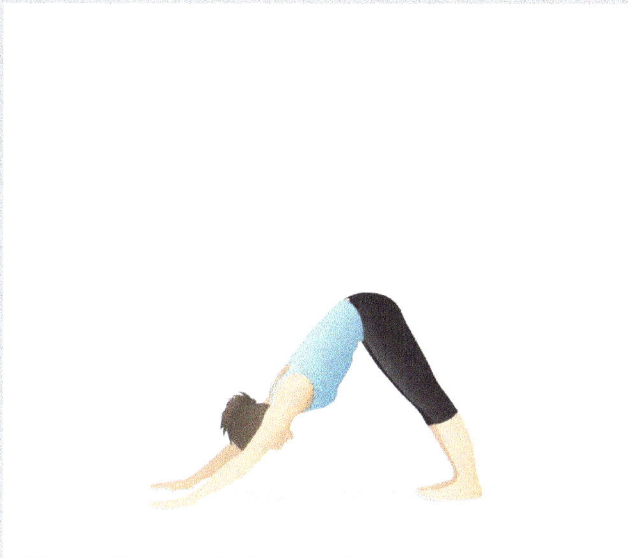

 This pose helps to stop hair from falling out and reduces stress relief. To do this position you must lie down flat on the floor On your abdomen. Your feet should be placed, palms all down, and aligned to the shoulder. Lift your body up with your upper body, you will be supporting your body with your hands while your feet and hands are downward.

Pose 2 Forward down position.

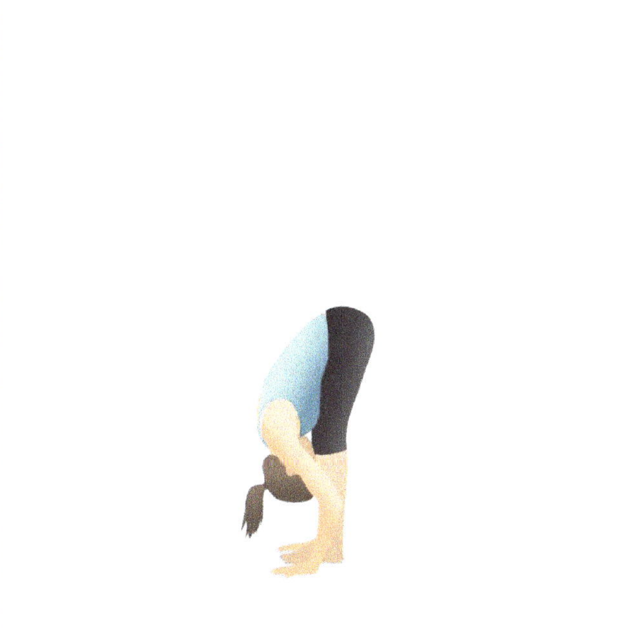

This pose is simple and easy. Simply stand straight and touch your toes, breathe in your pelvis out and bend forward. Slowly this pie gives oxygen to the brain and gives a signal to grow your hair.

Pose 3

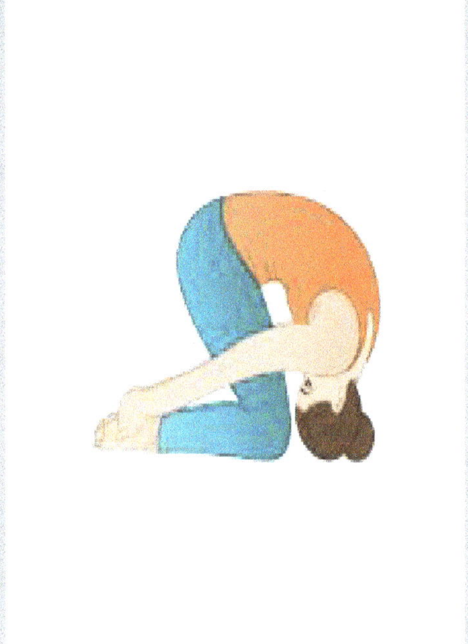

This next pose called Sasangasana could be complicated yet I will personally encourage you to take your time. Simply sit on your knees and lift your torso up. Then bend down so that your head rests on the floor. Stretch your hands behind you and hold your ankles. Breathe in and out and hold for at least 5 minutes. Do this pose every week in the morning and you will have rejuvenating hair. This pacific pose gives oxygen to the brain and hair follicles.

Closing chapter

To all my readers I hope that you can simply identify these facts by your own research. As you grow young to old to ageless to a greater higher being wishing you peace and love to all.

Copyright

I do not own **any** of these pictures except for the face pose ones of my niece. You can find these pictures (**Except for my niece!**) by simply searching them on google.com, thanks in advance!